EPI DIET FOOD LIST

2024

Managing Symptoms, Reducing Inflammation, and Savoring Flavor.
Includes a 21-Day Meal Plan of Delicious, Nutritious Recipes

DR. AMANDA SMITH

TABLE OF CONTENTS

Introduction 5

Chapter 1 8

WHAT YOU NEED TO KNOW ABOUT EPI 8

Understanding the Epi Diet..8

Benefits of Following the Epi Diet 8

How to Use This Book 10

Chapter 2 12

Epi Diet Basics..12

Principles of the Epi Diet...12

Macronutrient Ratios..14

Food Categories Allowed and Restricted...................15

Chapter 3 18

Epi Diet Food List..18

Fruits..18

Vegetables...22

Proteins 26

Grains and Carbohydrates...30

Fats and Oils..34

Beverages 38

Sweeteners..42

Condiments and Seasonings 47

Chapter 4 52

Recipes...52

Break Fast 52

Lunch...63

Dinner 76

Chapter 5 91

Meal Planning 91

    21 days meal plan...................................... 91

Chapter 6 97

Shopping Guide 97

    How to Shop for Epi Diet Foods................... 97

    Reading Labels and Identifying Epi Diet-Friendly Products 99

Chapter 7 102

Conclusion 102

INTRODUCTION

In today's fast-paced world, where various dietary trends constantly emerge, the Epi Diet stands out as a holistic approach to nutrition and overall well-being. Developed with the aim of optimizing health, vitality, and longevity, the Epi Diet focuses on consuming nutrient-dense foods that support the body's natural processes while minimizing inflammation and promoting metabolic flexibility.

The term "Epi Diet" is derived from "epigenetics," a field of science that explores how lifestyle factors, including diet, exercise, and environmental influences, can influence gene expression. By harnessing the power of epigenetics, the Epi Diet emphasizes the importance of food choices in shaping our health outcomes.

At its core, the Epi Diet emphasizes whole, minimally processed foods that are rich in essential nutrients and phytochemicals. By prioritizing quality over quantity, the Epi Diet encourages individuals to focus on the nutritional value of their food rather than simply counting calories or macronutrients.

One of the key principles of the Epi Diet is balance. Rather than advocating for strict dietary restrictions or deprivation, the Epi Diet emphasizes a balanced approach to eating, where all food groups have a place within the diet.

However, the emphasis is placed on choosing foods that nourish the body and support optimal health.

Central to the Epi Diet is the concept of metabolic flexibility. This refers to the body's ability to efficiently switch between different fuel sources, such as carbohydrates, fats, and ketones, depending on metabolic demands. By incorporating a variety of nutrient-dense foods into the diet, the Epi Diet promotes metabolic flexibility, which may help improve energy levels, enhance cognitive function, and support overall metabolic health.

In this comprehensive guide to the Epi Diet Food List 2024, we will delve into the specific foods that are recommended and restricted on the Epi Diet. From fruits and vegetables to proteins, fats, and carbohydrates, we will provide you with a detailed overview of the foods that can help you thrive on the Epi Diet. Additionally, we will offer practical tips for meal planning, shopping, dining out, and traveling while following the Epi Diet, as well as address common questions and concerns.

Whether you are looking to optimize your health, manage chronic conditions, or simply adopt a more balanced approach to eating, the Epi Diet offers a flexible and sustainable framework that can be tailored to individual preferences and needs. By incorporating nutrient-dense foods and promoting metabolic flexibility, the Epi Diet empowers individuals to take control of their health and unlock their full potential for vitality and well-being.

CHAPTER 1

WHAT YOU NEED TO KNOW ABOUT EPI

Understanding the Epi Diet

The Epi Diet, short for Epigenetic Diet, is a nutritional approach grounded in the principles of epigenetics, which explores how lifestyle factors, including diet, can influence gene expression and health outcomes. By emphasizing whole, nutrient-dense foods and promoting metabolic flexibility, the Epi Diet aims to optimize health, vitality, and longevity.

Benefits of Following the Epi Diet

Improved Health: The Epi Diet focuses on consuming foods rich in essential nutrients, antioxidants, and phytochemicals, which support overall health and well-being. By nourishing the body with high-quality foods, individuals may experience improvements in energy levels, immune function, and disease prevention.

Weight Management: Unlike fad diets that rely on strict calorie counting or food restrictions, the Epi Diet promotes a balanced approach to eating that emphasizes the quality of food over quantity. By prioritizing nutrient-dense foods and supporting metabolic flexibility, the Epi Diet may help individuals achieve and maintain a healthy weight.

Enhanced Metabolic Flexibility: Metabolic flexibility refers to the body's ability to efficiently switch between different fuel sources, such as carbohydrates, fats, and ketones, depending on metabolic demands. By incorporating a variety of nutrient-dense foods into the diet, the Epi Diet promotes metabolic flexibility, which may improve energy levels, enhance cognitive function, and support overall metabolic health.

Reduced Inflammation: Chronic inflammation is linked to various health conditions, including heart disease, diabetes, and autoimmune disorders. The Epi Diet emphasizes foods that have anti-inflammatory properties, such as fruits, vegetables, and healthy fats, while minimizing pro-inflammatory foods, such as processed foods and refined sugars. By reducing inflammation, individuals may experience improvements in overall health and well-being.

Long-Term Sustainability: Unlike restrictive diets that are difficult to maintain over the long term, the Epi Diet offers a flexible and sustainable approach to eating. By focusing on whole, minimally processed foods and incorporating a variety of flavors and textures, the Epi Diet can be adapted to individual preferences and needs, making it easier to stick with over time.

How to Use This Book

This book is designed to be your comprehensive guide to navigating the Epi Diet Food List 2024.

Educational Foundation:

Begin by immersing yourself in the introductory sections of the book. Gain a thorough understanding of the Epi Diet's principles, benefits, and how it aligns with your health goals.

Explore the Food Lists:

Dive into the detailed breakdown of Epi Diet-approved and restricted foods. Organized by food groups, these lists serve as your reference when planning meals and creating your grocery shopping list.

Meal Planning and Recipes:

Discover sample meal plans tailored to the Epi Diet, along with a plethora of recipe ideas and cooking suggestions. This section is invaluable for crafting nutritious and delicious meals that adhere to the Epi Diet guidelines.

Shopping Guide:

Learn essential tips for navigating the grocery store aisles with ease. Understand how to identify Epi Diet-friendly products, read food labels effectively, and make informed choices that align with your dietary preferences.

Dining Out and Traveling:

Gain insights into dining out at restaurants while adhering to the Epi Diet principles. Additionally, find strategies for maintaining your dietary goals while traveling, ensuring that you can stay on track regardless of your location.

By leveraging the information and resources provided within this book, you can effectively implement the Epi Diet into your lifestyle. Whether your aim is to manage chronic conditions, improve energy levels, or simply adopt a more balanced approach to eating, this book equips you with the knowledge and tools necessary to achieve your health and wellness goals.

CHAPTER 2

EPI DIET BASICS

Principles of the Epi Diet

Nutrient-Dense Foods: The Epi Diet emphasizes the consumption of nutrient-dense foods that provide a wide array of essential vitamins, minerals, antioxidants, and phytochemicals. These foods support overall health and well-being by nourishing the body at a cellular level.

Whole Foods: Central to the Epi Diet is the inclusion of whole, minimally processed foods. By prioritizing foods in their natural state, the diet ensures that individuals receive maximum nutritional benefit without the added sugars, unhealthy fats, and artificial additives often found in processed foods.

Balanced Macronutrients: The Epi Diet encourages a balanced intake of macronutrients, including carbohydrates, proteins, and fats. Rather than focusing on strict macronutrient ratios, the diet emphasizes the importance of incorporating a variety of nutrient-dense foods from each macronutrient category.

Metabolic Flexibility: Metabolic flexibility is a key principle of the Epi Diet. The diet promotes the body's ability to efficiently switch between different fuel sources, such as carbohydrates, fats, and ketones, depending on metabolic demands. By incorporating a diverse range of foods into the diet, individuals can support metabolic flexibility and optimize overall metabolic health.

Inflammation Reduction: Chronic inflammation is associated with a range of health conditions, including heart disease, diabetes, and autoimmune disorders. The Epi Diet focuses on reducing inflammation by emphasizing anti-inflammatory foods, such as fruits, vegetables, and healthy fats, while minimizing pro-inflammatory foods, such as processed foods and refined sugars.

Individualization: The Epi Diet recognizes that individual nutritional needs may vary based on factors such as age, gender, activity level, and health status. Therefore, the diet encourages individuals to personalize their food choices and dietary approach according to their unique preferences and needs.

Long-Term Sustainability: Unlike fad diets that promote quick fixes or extreme restrictions, the Epi Diet prioritizes long-term sustainability and lifestyle changes. By providing a flexible framework that can be adapted to individual preferences and circumstances, the diet promotes adherence and encourages lasting health improvements.

By adhering to these principles, individuals can harness the power of the Epi Diet to optimize their health, vitality, and longevity, while enjoying a diverse and delicious array of nutrient-dense foods.

Macronutrient Ratios

The Epi Diet does not prescribe rigid macronutrient ratios like some other dietary approaches. Instead, it emphasizes the importance of balance and variety in macronutrient intake. However, individuals following the Epi Diet typically aim for a balanced distribution of macronutrients to support overall health and well-being.

Carbohydrates: Carbohydrates are an essential source of energy for the body. The Epi Diet encourages the consumption of complex carbohydrates from whole, minimally processed sources such as fruits, vegetables, legumes, and whole grains. These foods provide fiber, vitamins, and minerals, and are often prioritized over refined carbohydrates like white bread and sugary snacks.

Proteins: Protein is crucial for building and repairing tissues, supporting immune function, and maintaining muscle mass. The Epi Diet includes a variety of protein sources such as lean meats, poultry, fish, eggs, dairy products, legumes, nuts, and seeds. Individuals following the Epi Diet aim to include adequate protein in their meals to support overall health and satiety.

Fats: Healthy fats play a vital role in hormone production, brain function, and nutrient absorption. The Epi Diet emphasizes the consumption of monounsaturated and polyunsaturated fats found in foods like avocados, nuts, seeds, olive oil, and fatty fish. Saturated fats from sources like coconut oil and grass-fed butter are also included in moderation, while trans fats are avoided.

While there is no one-size-fits-all macronutrient ratio prescribed by the Epi Diet, individuals may experiment with different ratios to find what works best for their bodies and goals. Some may thrive on a higher-carbohydrate approach, while others may prefer a higher-fat or balanced approach. Ultimately, the key is to prioritize nutrient-dense foods and listen to your body's hunger and satiety cues to achieve optimal health and well-being.

Food Categories Allowed and Restricted

Food Categories Allowed:

- Fruits (e.g., apples, berries, oranges)
- Vegetables (e.g., spinach, broccoli, carrots)
- Lean meats (e.g., chicken breast, turkey, lean cuts of beef)

- Fish and seafood (e.g., salmon, tuna, shrimp)
- Eggs
- Dairy products (e.g., Greek yogurt, cottage cheese, cheese)
- Legumes (e.g., lentils, chickpeas, black beans)
- Whole grains (e.g., quinoa, brown rice, oats)
- Nuts and seeds (e.g., almonds, walnuts, chia seeds)
- Healthy fats and oils (e.g., olive oil, avocado, flaxseed oil)
- Herbs and spices (e.g., basil, turmeric, cinnamon)
- Tea (e.g., green tea, herbal tea)
- Coffee (in moderation)
- Non-starchy vegetables (e.g., kale, cauliflower, bell peppers)
- Fermented foods (e.g., yogurt, kimchi, sauerkraut)
- Natural sweeteners (e.g., honey, maple syrup, stevia)
- Dark chocolate (in moderation)
- Seaweed and algae (e.g., nori, spirulina)
- Nutritional yeast
- Coconut products (e.g., coconut milk, coconut oil, unsweetened coconut flakes)

Food Categories Restricted:

- Processed foods (e.g., packaged snacks, frozen meals)

- Refined sugars (e.g., white sugar, high-fructose corn syrup)
- Artificial sweeteners (e.g., aspartame, sucralose)
- Trans fats (e.g., hydrogenated oils, margarine)
- Highly processed grains (e.g., white bread, white rice)
- Fast food (e.g., burgers, fries, pizza)
- Sugary beverages (e.g., soda, fruit juices, energy drinks)
- Deep-fried foods
- Processed meats (e.g., bacon, sausage, deli meats)
- Artificial additives and preservatives (e.g., MSG, artificial colors)
- Excessive alcohol
- High-sodium foods (e.g., processed snacks, canned soups)
- Margarine and other hydrogenated fats
- Sugary desserts and pastries (e.g., cakes, cookies, doughnuts)
- Sugary cereals
- White flour products (e.g., white bread, pasta)
- Sweetened condiments (e.g., ketchup, barbecue sauce)
- Artificial flavorings and colorings
- Processed cheeses
- Microwave popcorn with artificial additives

CHAPTER 3

EPI DIET FOOD LIST

Fruits

1. Apples
2. Bananas
3. Oranges
4. Strawberries
5. Blueberries
6. Raspberries
7. Blackberries
8. Grapes
9. Pineapple
10. Mangoes
11. Papaya
12. Kiwi
13. Watermelon
14. Cantaloupe
15. Honeydew melon
16. Peaches
17. Nectarines
18. Plums
19. Apricots
20. Cherries
21. Pears

22. Grapefruit

23. Lemon

24. Lime

25. Cranberries

26. Pomegranate

27. Guava

28. Passion fruit

29. Dragon fruit

30. Fig

31. Lychee

32. Kiwifruit

33. Tangerines

34. Clementines

35. Pomelo

36. Persimmons

37. Starfruit

38. Mulberries

39. Boysenberries

40. Goji berries

41. Loganberries

42. Elderberries

43. Kumquats

44. Plantains

45. Dates

46. Figs

47. Avocado (technically a fruit)
48. Jackfruit
49. Cranberries
50. Lingonberries
51. Marionberries
52. Olallieberries
53. Pepino
54. Prickly pear
55. Soursop
56. Ugli fruit
57. Yuzu
58. Blood orange
59. Cara Cara orange
60. Tamarillo
61. Tamarind
62. Sapote
63. Persimmon
64. Cape gooseberry
65. Feijoa
66. Acai berry
67. Acerola
68. Ackee
69. Agave
70. Ambarella
71. Aronia berry

72. Bael fruit

73. Barbadine

74. Barberry

75. Bilberry

76. Black sapote

77. Breadfruit

78. Buddha's hand

79. Cactus pear

80. Carambola

81. Chayote

82. Cloudberry

83. Cocona

84. Cupuacu

85. Durian

86. Elephant apple

87. Finger lime

88. Gac

89. Goldenberry

90. Hala fruit

91. Jujube

92. Longan

93. Lucuma

94. Miracle fruit

95. Monstera deliciosa

96. Noni

97. Pawpaw

98. Pepino melon

99. Persimmon

100.   Pitahaya (also known as dragon fruit)

Vegetables

1. Spinach

2. Kale

3. Broccoli

4. Cauliflower

5. Carrots

6. Bell peppers

7. Tomatoes

8. Cucumbers

9. Zucchini

10. Eggplant

11. Brussels sprouts

12. Asparagus

13. Celery

14. Green beans

15. Peas

16. Onions

17. Garlic

18. Mushrooms

19. Lettuce (various types like romaine, iceberg, arugula)

20. Cabbage (green, red, savoy)

21. Radishes

22. Beetroot

23. Swiss chard

24. Collard greens

25. Bok choy

26. Snow peas

27. Sugar snap peas

28. Artichokes

29. Fennel

30. Leeks

31. Parsnips

32. Turnips

33. Rutabaga

34. Watercress

35. Okra

36. Kohlrabi

37. Radicchio

38. Endive

39. Escarole

40. Mustard greens

41. Dandelion greens

42. Chicory

43. Chinese cabbage

44. Jicama

45. Sprouts (alfalfa, mung bean, broccoli)

46. Pumpkin

47. Butternut squash

48. Acorn squash

49. Spaghetti squash

50. Kabocha squash

51. Hubbard squash

52. Delicata squash

53. Sweet potatoes

54. Yukon gold potatoes

55. Red potatoes

56. Fingerling potatoes

57. New potatoes

58. Purple potatoes

59. Jerusalem artichoke (sunchokes)

60. Celeriac

61. Chinese broccoli

62. Chinese cabbage

63. Chinese eggplant

64. Chinese long beans

65. Chinese mustard greens

66. Yu choy

67. Gai choy

68. Bitter melon

69. Malabar spinach

70. Yardlong beans

71. Tatsoi

72. Chayote

73. Taro

74. Bamboo shoots

75. Lotus root

76. Napa cabbage

77. Daikon radish

78. Winter melon

79. Water spinach

80. Winged beans

81. Vietnamese coriander

82. Thai eggplant

83. Thai basil

84. Thai chilies

85. Thai pea eggplant

86. Thai pumpkin

87. Thai spinach

88. Thai sweet basil

89. Thai lime leaves

90. Thai morning glory

91. Thai bean sprouts

92. Thai yardlong beans

93. Thai galangal

94. Thai lemongrass

95. Thai kaffir lime
96. Thai holy basil
97. Thai snake beans
98. Thai winged beans
99. Thai shallots
100. Thai garlic

Proteins

1. Chicken breast
2. Turkey breast
3. Lean beef (such as sirloin or tenderloin)
4. Pork tenderloin
5. Lean cuts of lamb
6. Bison
7. Venison
8. Veal
9. Rabbit
10. Duck breast
11. Goose breast
12. Quail
13. Pheasant
14. Ostrich
15. Elk
16. Emu
17. Kangaroo

18. Buffalo
19. Cornish game hen
20. Chicken thighs (skinless)
21. Chicken drumsticks (skinless)
22. Ground chicken
23. Ground turkey
24. Ground beef (lean)
25. Ground pork (lean)
26. Ground lamb (lean)
27. Ground bison
28. Ground venison
29. Ground veal
30. Ground rabbit
31. Ground duck
32. Ground goose
33. Ground quail
34. Ground ostrich
35. Ground elk
36. Ground emu
37. Ground kangaroo
38. Ground buffalo
39. Eggs (chicken)
40. Eggs (duck)
41. Eggs (quail)
42. Eggs (goose)

43. Eggs (turkey)

44. Eggs (ostrich)

45. Eggs (emu)

46. Eggs (pheasant)

47. Eggs (guinea fowl)

48. Eggs (pigeon)

49. Eggs (partridge)

50. Eggs (rhea)

51. Eggs (snake)

52. Eggs (reptile)

53. Eggs (frog)

54. Eggs (insect)

55. Eggs (fish)

56. Eggs (shellfish)

57. Salmon

58. Trout

59. Tuna

60. Cod

61. Halibut

62. Haddock

63. Snapper

64. Sea bass

65. Mahi-mahi

66. Swordfish

67. Tilapia

68. Catfish

69. Sardines

70. Anchovies

71. Mackerel

72. Herring

73. Perch

74. Pollock

75. Flounder

76. Sole

77. Arctic char

78. Bass

79. Carp

80. Eel

81. Monkfish

82. Shark

83. Sturgeon

84. Wahoo

85. Barracuda

86. Grouper

87. Tilefish

88. Amberjack

89. Kingfish

90. Marlin

91. Pompano

92. Rockfish

93. Wrasse

94. Bluefish

95. Drum

96. Triggerfish

97. Jackfish

98. Opah

99. Saury

100. Black cod

Grains and Carbohydrates

1. Quinoa

2. Brown rice

3. Basmati rice

4. Jasmine rice

5. Wild rice

6. Black rice

7. Red rice

8. Forbidden rice

9. Bulgur

10. Farro

11. Barley

12. Millet

13. Buckwheat

14. Amaranth

15. Teff

16. Sorghum

17. Spelt

18. Kamut

19. Freekeh

20. Whole wheat pasta

21. Whole grain couscous

22. Oats

23. Steel-cut oats

24. Rolled oats

25. Oat bran

26. Oat flour

27. Whole wheat flour

28. Buckwheat flour

29. Barley flour

30. Spelt flour

31. Rye flour

32. Kamut flour

33. Millet flour

34. Teff flour

35. Sorghum flour

36. Coconut flour

37. Almond flour

38. Hazelnut flour

39. Chestnut flour

40. Chickpea flour (besan)

41. Lentil flour
42. Fava bean flour
43. Pea flour
44. Sorghum flour
45. Tapioca flour
46. Arrowroot flour
47. Potato flour
48. Cornmeal
49. Polenta
50. Grits
51. Corn flour
52. Hominy
53. Buckwheat groats
54. Bulgur
55. Wheat berries
56. Corn tortillas
57. Whole wheat tortillas
58. Sprouted grain bread
59. Ezekiel bread
60. Rye bread
61. Whole grain bread
62. Spelt bread
63. Kamut bread
64. Buckwheat bread
65. Oat bread

66. Barley bread

67. Millet bread

68. Quinoa bread

69. Brown rice cakes

70. Whole grain crackers

71. Popcorn

72. Whole wheat pita bread

73. Whole wheat naan bread

74. Whole grain bagels

75. Whole grain English muffins

76. Whole grain wraps

77. Whole grain cereal

78. Muesli

79. Granola

80. Bran flakes

81. Wheat bran

82. Wheat germ

83. Corn flakes

84. Rice cakes

85. Buckwheat pancakes

86. Oat pancakes

87. Whole wheat pancakes

88. Buckwheat waffles

89. Oat waffles

90. Whole wheat waffles

91. Sorghum syrup

92. Barley malt syrup

93. Brown rice syrup

94. Maple syrup

95. Date syrup

96. Molasses

97. Honey

98. Agave nectar

99. Coconut sugar

100. Palm sugar

Fats and Oils

1. Olive oil

2. Avocado oil

3. Coconut oil

4. Flaxseed oil

5. Walnut oil

6. Hemp seed oil

7. Sesame oil

8. Sunflower oil

9. Safflower oil

10. Canola oil

11. Peanut oil

12. Grapeseed oil

13. Almond oil

14. Pistachio oil
15. Macadamia nut oil
16. Pecan oil
17. Hazelnut oil
18. Cashew oil
19. Pine nut oil
20. Pumpkin seed oil
21. Sardine oil
22. Mackerel oil
23. Cod liver oil
24. Krill oil
25. Fish oil
26. Emu oil
27. Tallow
28. Lard
29. Duck fat
30. Ghee (clarified butter)
31. Butter
32. Margarine (in moderation and preferably plant-based)
33. Shortening
34. Palm oil
35. Palm kernel oil
36. Rice bran oil
37. Corn oil
38. Soybean oil

39. Flaxseeds

40. Chia seeds

41. Hemp seeds

42. Pumpkin seeds

43. Sunflower seeds

44. Sesame seeds

45. Poppy seeds

46. Pine nuts

47. Walnuts

48. Almonds

49. Pecans

50. Cashews

51. Macadamia nuts

52. Brazil nuts

53. Hazelnuts

54. Pistachios

55. Coconuts

56. Coconut butter

57. Coconut cream

58. Coconut milk

59. Coconut flakes

60. Avocado

61. Olives

62. Dark chocolate (in moderation)

63. Cacao nibs

64. Cocoa powder

65. MCT oil (medium-chain triglyceride oil)

66. Algal oil

67. Flaxseeds

68. Chia seeds

69. Hemp seeds

70. Sunflower seeds

71. Pumpkin seeds

72. Sesame seeds

73. Poppy seeds

74. Pine nuts

75. Walnuts

76. Almonds

77. Pecans

78. Cashews

79. Macadamia nuts

80. Brazil nuts

81. Hazelnuts

82. Pistachios

83. Chestnuts

84. Butternuts

85. Hulled sunflower seeds

86. Hulled pumpkin seeds

87. Flaxseed meal

88. Chia seed meal

89. Hemp seed meal

90. Sunflower seed meal

91. Pumpkin seed meal

92. Sesame seed meal

93. Walnut meal

94. Almond meal

95. Pecan meal

96. Cashew meal

97. Macadamia nut meal

98. Brazil nut meal

99. Hazelnut meal

100. Pistachio meal

Beverages

1. Water

2. Sparkling water

3. Mineral water

4. Flavored water (unsweetened)

5. Herbal tea (such as chamomile, peppermint, or rooibos)

6. Green tea

7. Black tea

8. White tea

9. Oolong tea

10. Matcha tea

11. Yerba mate

12. Ginger tea

13. Turmeric tea

14. Lemon water (with or without honey)

15. Lime water (with or without honey)

16. Cucumber water

17. Fruit-infused water (with berries, citrus, or cucumber)

18. Coconut water

19. Almond milk (unsweetened)

20. Soy milk (unsweetened)

21. Oat milk (unsweetened)

22. Rice milk (unsweetened)

23. Cashew milk (unsweetened)

24. Hemp milk (unsweetened)

25. Flax milk (unsweetened)

26. Macadamia nut milk (unsweetened)

27. Walnut milk (unsweetened)

28. Hazelnut milk (unsweetened)

29. Pistachio milk (unsweetened)

30. Pecan milk (unsweetened)

31. Brazil nut milk (unsweetened)

32. Sunflower seed milk (unsweetened)

33. Pumpkin seed milk (unsweetened)

34. Sesame seed milk (unsweetened)

35. Pine nut milk (unsweetened)

36. Quinoa milk (unsweetened)

37. Amaranth milk (unsweetened)

38. Millet milk (unsweetened)

39. Barley milk (unsweetened)

40. Buckwheat milk (unsweetened)

41. Chia seed milk (unsweetened)

42. Hemp seed milk (unsweetened)

43. Coconut milk (unsweetened)

44. Coconut cream

45. Nut-based hot chocolate (unsweetened)

46. Carob-based hot chocolate (unsweetened)

47. Chicory root coffee (unsweetened)

48. Dandelion root coffee (unsweetened)

49. Mushroom coffee (unsweetened)

50. Beetroot latte (unsweetened)

51. Turmeric latte (unsweetened)

52. Matcha latte (unsweetened)

53. Ginger turmeric latte (unsweetened)

54. Golden milk (unsweetened)

55. Protein shakes (made with unsweetened protein powder)

56. Vegetable juice (such as tomato, carrot, or beet)

57. Fruit juice (unsweetened and diluted with water)

58. Green juice (made with leafy greens and other vegetables)

59. Wheatgrass juice

60. Aloe vera juice

61. Kombucha (unsweetened or lightly sweetened)

62. Fermented coconut water

63. Fermented tea (such as kombucha or Jun)

64. Kvass (fermented beverage made from rye bread)

65. Switchel (apple cider vinegar-based beverage)

66. Herbal tonics (such as fire cider or elderberry syrup)

67. Electrolyte drinks (without added sugars)

68. Bone broth (unsweetened)

69. Vegetable broth (unsweetened)

70. Miso soup (unsweetened)

71. Seaweed broth (unsweetened)

72. Coconut milk-based soup (unsweetened)

73. Almond milk-based soup (unsweetened)

74. Vegetable smoothies (without added sugars)

75. Fruit smoothies (unsweetened and made with whole fruits)

76. Green smoothies (made with leafy greens and other vegetables)

77. Protein smoothies (made with unsweetened protein powder)

78. Avocado smoothies (unsweetened)

79. Chia seed smoothies (unsweetened)

80. Hemp seed smoothies (unsweetened)

81. Coconut water smoothies (unsweetened)

82. Nut milk smoothies (unsweetened)

83. Herbal smoothies (unsweetened)

84. Vegetable milkshakes (unsweetened)

85. Fruit milkshakes (unsweetened and made with whole fruits)

86. Nut milk milkshakes (unsweetened)

87. Seed milk milkshakes (unsweetened)

88. Coconut milk milkshakes (unsweetened)

89. Herbal milkshakes (unsweetened)

90. Iced herbal tea (unsweetened)

91. Iced green tea (unsweetened)

92. Iced black tea (unsweetened)

93. Iced white tea (unsweetened)

94. Iced oolong tea (unsweetened)

95. Iced matcha tea (unsweetened)

96. Iced yerba mate (unsweetened)

97. Iced ginger tea (unsweetened)

98. Iced turmeric tea (unsweetened)

99. Iced lemon water (with or without honey)

100.   Iced lime water (with or without honey)

Sweeteners

1. Honey

2. Maple syrup

3. Agave nectar

4. Date syrup

5. Molasses

6. Coconut sugar

7. Brown rice syrup

8. Barley malt syrup

9. Blackstrap molasses

10. Stevia

11. Monk fruit extract (luo han guo)

12. Erythritol

13. Xylitol

14. Allulose

15. Yacon syrup

16. Lucuma powder

17. Mesquite powder

18. Coconut nectar

19. Birch syrup

20. Sorghum syrup

21. Panela (unrefined whole cane sugar)

22. Rapadura (unrefined whole cane sugar)

23. Palm sugar

24. Date sugar

25. Fruit juice concentrate (unsweetened)

26. Grape molasses

27. Pomegranate molasses

28. Birch sugar (xylitol)

29. Maltitol

30. Dextrose

31. Fructose

32. Malt syrup

33. Rice malt syrup

34. Tapioca syrup

35. Sweet potato syrup

36. Stevia glycerite

37. Tagatose

38. Coconut palm sugar

39. Raw cane sugar

40. Muscovado sugar

41. Demerara sugar

42. Turbinado sugar

43. Golden syrup

44. Inulin

45. Chicory root syrup

46. Monk fruit sweetener

47. Date paste

48. Coconut syrup

49. Birch xylitol

50. Maltodextrin

51. Sorbitol

52. Mannitol

53. Isomalt

54. Glycyrrhizin (licorice root extract)
55. Mabinlin (a protein extracted from the African plant Capparis masaikai)
56. Brazzein (a protein found in the fruit of the West African plant Pentadiplandra brazzeana)
57. Thaumatin (a protein extracted from the fruit of the katemfe plant)
58. Neohesperidin dihydrochalcone (NHDC)
59. Luo han guo (monk fruit)
60. Soran fruit
61. Blue agave syrup
62. Cane sugar
63. Turbinado sugar
64. Evaporated cane juice
65. Granulated maple sugar
66. Palm syrup
67. High fructose corn syrup (HFCS) - in moderation and preferably in its natural form
68. Grape syrup
69. Date honey
70. Carob syrup
71. Coconut sap
72. Gula melaka (palm sugar from Southeast Asia)
73. Rapadura sugar
74. Palm jaggery

75. Birch sugar
76. Birch xylitol
77. Isomalt
78. Maltitol
79. Maltitol syrup
80. Polydextrose
81. Tagatose
82. Xylitol syrup
83. Erythritol syrup
84. Stevia leaf powder
85. Lucuma syrup
86. Maple sugar
87. Date syrup
88. Inulin syrup
89. Sorbitol syrup
90. Maltitol syrup
91. Maltodextrin syrup
92. Honey granules
93. Maple granules
94. Yacon powder
95. Coconut sugar granules
96. Date sugar
97. Inulin powder
98. Sorbitol powder
99. Maltitol powder

100. Xylitol powder

CONDIMENTS AND SEASONINGS

1. Salt (sea salt, Himalayan salt, kosher salt)
2. Black pepper
3. White pepper
4. Cayenne pepper
5. Paprika
6. Chili powder
7. Cumin
8. Coriander
9. Turmeric
10. Ginger (ground or fresh)
11. Cinnamon
12. Nutmeg
13. Allspice
14. Cloves
15. Cardamom
16. Mustard powder
17. Dried basil
18. Dried oregano
19. Dried thyme
20. Dried rosemary
21. Dried parsley
22. Dried dill

23. Dried cilantro
24. Dried mint
25. Dried sage
26. Dried marjoram
27. Dried tarragon
28. Dried bay leaves
29. Dried savory
30. Dried chives
31. Dried coriander leaves (cilantro)
32. Dried lemon peel
33. Dried orange peel
34. Dried lime peel
35. Dried grapefruit peel
36. Dried garlic powder
37. Dried onion powder
38. Dried shallots
39. Dried leeks
40. Dried scallions (green onions)
41. Dried celery flakes
42. Dried bell pepper flakes
43. Dried tomato flakes
44. Dried mushroom powder
45. Dried seaweed flakes
46. Dried lemon grass
47. Dried kaffir lime leaves

48. Dried galangal

49. Dried turmeric root

50. Dried ginger root

51. Dried fenugreek leaves

52. Dried curry leaves

53. Dried fenugreek seeds

54. Dried mustard seeds

55. Dried fennel seeds

56. Dried coriander seeds

57. Dried cumin seeds

58. Dried caraway seeds

59. Dried sesame seeds

60. Dried poppy seeds

61. Dried nigella seeds (black cumin)

62. Dried anise seeds

63. Dried dill seeds

64. Dried basil seeds

65. Dried marjoram seeds

66. Dried rosemary seeds

67. Dried thyme seeds

68. Dried savory seeds

69. Dried tarragon seeds

70. Dried mint seeds

71. Dried parsley seeds

72. Dried cilantro seeds (coriander)

73. Dried chia seeds

74. Dried sunflower seeds

75. Dried pumpkin seeds

76. Dried flax seeds

77. Dried hemp seeds

78. Dried quinoa seeds

79. Dried amaranth seeds

80. Dried sesame seeds

81. Dried sunflower seeds

82. Dried poppy seeds

83. Dried nigella seeds

84. Dried chia seeds

85. Dried mustard seeds

86. Dried fennel seeds

87. Dried caraway seeds

88. Dried fenugreek seeds

89. Dried cumin seeds

90. Dried coriander seeds

91. Dried cardamom seeds

92. Dried celery seeds

93. Dried anise seeds

94. Dried dill seeds

95. Dried fennel seeds

96. Dried basil seeds

97. Dried oregano seeds

98. Dried rosemary seeds

99. Dried thyme seeds

100. Dried tarragon seeds

CHAPTER 4

RECIPES

Break Fast

1. Avocado Breakfast Toast

- Prep Time: 10 mins
- Total Time: 10 mins
- Servings: 2

Ingredients:

- 2 slices of whole grain bread
- 1 ripe avocado
- 1 small tomato, sliced
- 2 boiled eggs, sliced
- Salt and pepper to taste
- Optional toppings: sliced radishes, microgreens, hot sauce

Directions:

- Toast the bread slices until golden brown.
- While the bread is toasting, mash the avocado in a bowl with a fork until smooth. Season with salt and pepper to taste.
- Spread the mashed avocado evenly onto the toasted bread slices.

- Top each slice with sliced tomato and boiled egg.
- Sprinkle with additional salt and pepper if desired, and add any optional toppings.
- Serve immediately.

Nutrition Facts (per serving):

- Calories: 275
- Fat: 14g
- Saturated fat: 2g
- Cholesterol: 186mg
- Sodium: 298mg
- Carbohydrate: 26g
- Fiber: 7g
- Sugars: 3g
- Protein: 14g
- Vitamin D: 50mcg
- Calcium: 97mg
- Iron: 2mg
- Potassium: 720mg

Other Ways to Enjoy:

Avocado Breakfast Wrap: Spread mashed avocado on a whole grain tortilla, add sliced tomato, boiled egg, and any other desired toppings. Roll up the tortilla tightly and enjoy as a portable breakfast.

Avocado Breakfast Bowl: Skip the bread and serve mashed avocado, sliced tomato, boiled egg, and any desired toppings in a bowl. Drizzle with a little olive oil and sprinkle with salt and pepper for a nutritious breakfast bowl option.

2. Greek Yogurt Parfait

- Prep Time: 10 mins
- Total Time: 10 mins
- Servings: 2

Ingredients:

- 1 cup plain Greek yogurt
- 1 tablespoon honey
- 1/2 cup fresh berries (such as strawberries, blueberries, or raspberries)
- 1/4 cup granola
- Optional toppings: sliced almonds, shredded coconut, chia seeds

Directions:

- In a bowl, mix together Greek yogurt and honey until well combined.
- In two serving glasses or bowls, layer the Greek yogurt mixture, fresh berries, and granola.

- Repeat the layers until all ingredients are used up, ending with a layer of granola on top.
- Sprinkle optional toppings such as sliced almonds, shredded coconut, or chia seeds over the parfait.
- Serve immediately.

Nutrition Facts (per serving):

- Calories: 250
- Fat: 6g
- Saturated fat: 1g
- Cholesterol: 10mg
- Sodium: 55mg
- Carbohydrate: 35g
- Fiber: 4g
- Sugars: 22g
- Protein: 16g
- Calcium: 184mg
- Iron: 1mg
- Potassium: 280mg

Other Ways to Enjoy:

Smoothie Bowl: Blend Greek yogurt, honey, and berries together until smooth. Pour into a bowl and top with granola, sliced fruit, and optional toppings for a refreshing smoothie bowl breakfast.

Breakfast Parfait Popsicles: Layer Greek yogurt, honey, berries, and granola in popsicle molds. Insert popsicle sticks and freeze until solid. Enjoy these nutritious and refreshing popsicles for breakfast on-the-go.

3. Vegetable Egg Muffins

- Prep Time: 15 mins
- Total Time: 30 mins
- Servings: 6

Ingredients:

- 6 large eggs
- 1/4 cup milk (or non-dairy milk)
- 1 cup chopped mixed vegetables (such as bell peppers, spinach, onions, tomatoes)
- 1/2 cup shredded cheese (such as cheddar, mozzarella, or feta)
- Salt and pepper to taste
- Cooking spray or olive oil for greasing muffin tin

Directions:

- Preheat the oven to 350°F (175°C). Grease a 6-cup muffin tin with cooking spray or olive oil.

- In a large mixing bowl, whisk together the eggs and milk until well combined. Season with salt and pepper.
- Stir in the chopped mixed vegetables and shredded cheese until evenly distributed.
- Pour the egg and vegetable mixture evenly into the prepared muffin tin, filling each cup about 3/4 full.
- Bake in the preheated oven for 15-20 minutes, or until the egg muffins are set and lightly golden on top.
- Remove from the oven and allow the egg muffins to cool for a few minutes before carefully removing them from the muffin tin.
- Serve warm as a nutritious breakfast option.

Nutrition Facts (per serving):

- Calories: 120
- Fat: 8g
- Saturated fat: 3g
- Cholesterol: 191mg
- Sodium: 150mg
- Carbohydrate: 3g
- Fiber: 1g
- Sugars: 2g
- Protein: 10g

- Vitamin D: 49IU
- Calcium: 104mg
- Iron: 1mg
- Potassium: 132mg

Other Ways to Enjoy:

Egg Muffin Breakfast Sandwich: Slice the egg muffins in half horizontally and layer with cooked turkey bacon or ham and sliced avocado for a delicious breakfast sandwich.

Egg Muffin Salad: Chop the egg muffins into bite-sized pieces and toss with mixed greens, cherry tomatoes, cucumber, and your favorite salad dressing for a satisfying breakfast salad option.

4. Quinoa Breakfast Bowl

- Prep Time: 5 mins
- Total Time: 20 mins
- Servings: 2

Ingredients:

- 1/2 cup quinoa, rinsed
- 1 cup water or vegetable broth
- 1/2 teaspoon cinnamon
- 1 tablespoon honey or maple syrup
- 1/2 cup Greek yogurt

- 1/2 cup mixed fresh fruit (such as berries, sliced banana, or diced apple)
- 2 tablespoons chopped nuts or seeds (such as almonds, walnuts, or pumpkin seeds)
- Optional toppings: shredded coconut, dried fruit, chia seeds

Directions:

- In a small saucepan, bring the water or vegetable broth to a boil. Add the quinoa and cinnamon, reduce heat to low, cover, and simmer for about 15 minutes, or until the quinoa is tender and the liquid is absorbed.
- Fluff the cooked quinoa with a fork and stir in the honey or maple syrup.
- Divide the cooked quinoa evenly between two bowls.
- Top each bowl with Greek yogurt, mixed fresh fruit, and chopped nuts or seeds.
- Sprinkle optional toppings such as shredded coconut, dried fruit, or chia seeds over the breakfast bowls.
- Serve warm or chilled, as desired.

Nutrition Facts (per serving):

- Calories: 310
- Fat: 9g
- Saturated fat: 1g
- Cholesterol: 3mg
- Sodium: 33mg
- Carbohydrate: 50g
- Fiber: 6g
- Sugars: 17g
- Protein: 11g
- Calcium: 102mg
- Iron: 3mg
- Potassium: 372mg

Other Ways to Enjoy:

Quinoa Breakfast Wrap: Wrap cooked quinoa, Greek yogurt, mixed fresh fruit, and chopped nuts or seeds in a whole grain tortilla for a portable breakfast option.

Quinoa Breakfast Smoothie: Blend cooked quinoa, Greek yogurt, mixed fresh fruit, and a splash of milk or fruit juice until smooth. Enjoy as a nutritious and filling breakfast smoothie.

5. Chia Seed Pudding

- Prep Time: 5 mins (plus chilling time)
- Total Time: 4 hours

- Servings: 2

Ingredients:

- 1/4 cup chia seeds
- 1 cup unsweetened almond milk (or any milk of choice)
- 1 tablespoon honey or maple syrup (optional)
- 1/2 teaspoon vanilla extract
- Fresh fruit for topping (such as sliced strawberries, blueberries, or kiwi)
- Nuts or seeds for topping (such as sliced almonds, chopped walnuts, or pumpkin seeds)
- Optional toppings: shredded coconut, cocoa nibs, granola

Directions:

- In a mixing bowl or jar, combine the chia seeds, almond milk, honey or maple syrup (if using), and vanilla extract. Stir well to combine.
- Cover the bowl or jar and refrigerate for at least 4 hours or overnight, until the chia pudding has thickened and set.
- Stir the chia pudding mixture well before serving to ensure that the chia seeds are evenly distributed.

- Divide the chia seed pudding into serving bowls or glasses.
- Top each serving with fresh fruit, nuts or seeds, and any optional toppings of your choice.
- Serve chilled and enjoy!

Nutrition Facts (per serving):

- Calories: 150
- Fat: 8g
- Saturated fat: 1g
- Cholesterol: 0mg
- Sodium: 80mg
- Carbohydrate: 15g
- Fiber: 10g
- Sugars: 4g
- Protein: 5g
- Calcium: 200mg
- Iron: 2mg
- Potassium: 160mg

Other Ways to Enjoy:

Chia Seed Breakfast Parfait: Layer chia seed pudding with Greek yogurt and fresh fruit in a glass or jar to create a delicious and visually appealing breakfast parfait.

Chia Seed Smoothie Bowl: Blend chia seed pudding with frozen fruit and a splash of almond milk until smooth. Pour into a bowl and top with additional fresh fruit, nuts, and seeds for a nutritious breakfast smoothie bowl.

Lunch

1. Quinoa Salad with Grilled Chicken

- Prep Time: 15 mins
- Total Time: 30 mins
- Servings: 2

Ingredients:

- 1/2 cup quinoa, rinsed
- 1 cup water or vegetable broth
- 2 small chicken breasts, boneless and skinless
- 1 tablespoon olive oil
- Salt and pepper to taste
- 2 cups mixed salad greens (such as spinach, arugula, or kale)
- 1/2 cup cherry tomatoes, halved
- 1/2 cucumber, sliced
- 1/4 cup sliced red onion
- 1/4 cup crumbled feta cheese
- 2 tablespoons balsamic vinaigrette dressing

Directions:

- In a small saucepan, bring the water or vegetable broth to a boil. Add the quinoa, reduce heat to low, cover, and simmer for about 15 minutes, or until the quinoa is tender and the liquid is absorbed. Fluff with a fork and set aside.
- Preheat a grill or grill pan over medium-high heat. Brush the chicken breasts with olive oil and season with salt and pepper.
- Grill the chicken breasts for 6-8 minutes per side, or until cooked through and no longer pink in the center. Remove from the grill and let rest for a few minutes before slicing.
- In a large mixing bowl, combine the cooked quinoa, mixed salad greens, cherry tomatoes, cucumber, red onion, and crumbled feta cheese. Toss with balsamic vinaigrette dressing until evenly coated.
- Divide the quinoa salad between two plates and top each with sliced grilled chicken.
- Serve immediately and enjoy!

Nutrition Facts (per serving):

- Calories: 390
- Fat: 16g

- Saturated fat: 4g
- Cholesterol: 90mg
- Sodium: 330mg
- Carbohydrate: 29g
- Fiber: 5g
- Sugars: 5g
- Protein: 32g
- Vitamin A: 110%
- Vitamin C: 40%
- Calcium: 15%
- Iron: 20%

Other Ways to Enjoy:

Quinoa Salad Wrap: Spoon the quinoa salad onto whole grain tortillas, add sliced grilled chicken, and wrap tightly for a portable and satisfying lunch option.

Quinoa Salad Bowl: Serve the quinoa salad in bowls and top with sliced avocado, roasted chickpeas, and a drizzle of tahini dressing for a hearty and nutritious grain bowl.

2. Mediterranean Chickpea Salad

- Prep Time: 15 mins
- Total Time: 15 mins
- Servings: 2

Ingredients:

- 1 can (15 ounces) chickpeas, drained and rinsed
- 1 cup cherry tomatoes, halved
- 1/2 cucumber, diced
- 1/4 red onion, thinly sliced
- 1/4 cup Kalamata olives, pitted and halved
- 1/4 cup crumbled feta cheese
- 2 tablespoons chopped fresh parsley
- 2 tablespoons extra virgin olive oil
- 1 tablespoon lemon juice
- 1 teaspoon dried oregano
- Salt and pepper to taste

Directions:

- In a large mixing bowl, combine the chickpeas, cherry tomatoes, cucumber, red onion, Kalamata olives, crumbled feta cheese, and chopped fresh parsley.
- Drizzle extra virgin olive oil and lemon juice over the salad. Sprinkle with dried oregano, salt, and pepper.
- Toss the salad gently until all ingredients are evenly coated with the dressing and seasonings.
- Divide the Mediterranean chickpea salad between two plates or bowls.

- Serve immediately as a delicious and nutritious lunch option.

Nutrition Facts (per serving):

- Calories: 320
- Fat: 18g
- Saturated fat: 4g
- Cholesterol: 13mg
- Sodium: 430mg
- Carbohydrate: 32g
- Fiber: 9g
- Sugars: 6g
- Protein: 11g
- Vitamin A: 25%
- Vitamin C: 35%
- Calcium: 15%
- Iron: 25%

Other Ways to Enjoy:

Mediterranean Chickpea Wrap: Spoon the chickpea salad onto whole grain wraps, add a handful of mixed greens, and roll tightly for a satisfying and portable lunch wrap.

Mediterranean Chickpea Pita Pocket: Fill whole wheat pita pockets with the chickpea salad, sliced cucumber, and a dollop of Greek yogurt or tzatziki sauce for a quick and flavorful lunch option.

3. Salmon and Quinoa Stuffed Bell Peppers

- Prep Time: 20 mins
- Total Time: 50 mins
- Servings: 2

Ingredients:

- 2 large bell peppers (any color), halved and seeds removed
- 2 (4-ounce) salmon fillets
- 1/2 cup quinoa, rinsed
- 1 cup water or vegetable broth
- 1 tablespoon olive oil
- 1/2 onion, diced
- 1 garlic clove, minced
- 1/2 cup diced tomatoes (fresh or canned)
- 1/4 cup chopped fresh parsley
- Salt and pepper to taste
- Optional toppings: grated Parmesan cheese, sliced green onions

Directions:

- Preheat the oven to 375°F (190°C). Place the bell pepper halves cut side up on a baking sheet lined with parchment paper.

- Season the salmon fillets with salt and pepper, then place them skin-side down on the baking sheet alongside the bell peppers.

- Roast in the preheated oven for 20-25 minutes, or until the salmon is cooked through and the bell peppers are slightly softened.

- While the salmon and bell peppers are roasting, cook the quinoa. In a small saucepan, bring the water or vegetable broth to a boil. Add the quinoa, reduce heat to low, cover, and simmer for about 15 minutes, or until the quinoa is tender and the liquid is absorbed. Fluff with a fork and set aside.

- In a skillet, heat the olive oil over medium heat. Add the diced onion and cook until softened, about 5 minutes. Add the minced garlic and cook for an additional minute.

- Stir in the diced tomatoes and cooked quinoa. Cook for another 2-3 minutes, then remove from heat. Stir in the chopped fresh parsley and season with salt and pepper to taste.

- Once the salmon and bell peppers are done roasting, remove them from the oven. Use a fork to flake the salmon into bite-sized pieces.
- Spoon the quinoa mixture into each bell pepper half, then top with flaked salmon.
- Optional: Sprinkle grated Parmesan cheese and sliced green onions over the stuffed bell peppers.
- Return the stuffed bell peppers to the oven and bake for an additional 5-10 minutes, or until heated through.
- Serve warm and enjoy!

Nutrition Facts (per serving):

- Calories: 380
- Fat: 15g
- Saturated fat: 2.5g
- Cholesterol: 60mg
- Sodium: 260mg
- Carbohydrate: 32g
- Fiber: 5g
- Sugars: 7g
- Protein: 30g
- Vitamin A: 80%
- Vitamin C: 220%
- Calcium: 6%

- Iron: 20%

Other Ways to Enjoy:

Salmon and Quinoa Salad: Flake the cooked salmon and mix with cooked quinoa, diced bell peppers, cucumber, cherry tomatoes, and a lemon vinaigrette dressing for a refreshing and protein-packed salad.

Salmon and Quinoa Lettuce Wraps: Use large lettuce leaves (such as romaine or butter lettuce) as wraps and fill them with flaked salmon, cooked quinoa, diced avocado, and a drizzle of tahini sauce for a light and nutritious lunch option.

4. Turkey and Vegetable Stir-Fry

- Prep Time: 15 mins
- Total Time: 25 mins
- Servings: 2

Ingredients:

- 8 ounces turkey breast, thinly sliced
- 2 tablespoons soy sauce (reduced-sodium)
- 1 tablespoon olive oil
- 2 cloves garlic, minced
- 1 teaspoon grated fresh ginger
- 1 bell pepper, thinly sliced

- 1 cup broccoli florets
- 1 cup snow peas
- 1 carrot, julienned
- 1/4 cup low-sodium chicken or vegetable broth
- 2 green onions, thinly sliced
- Sesame seeds for garnish (optional)
- Cooked quinoa or brown rice for serving

Directions:

- In a small bowl, marinate the sliced turkey breast in soy sauce for about 10 minutes.
- In a large skillet or wok, heat olive oil over medium-high heat. Add minced garlic and grated ginger, stirring constantly for about 30 seconds until fragrant.
- Add marinated turkey slices to the skillet and cook until browned and cooked through, about 3-4 minutes. Remove turkey from the skillet and set aside.
- In the same skillet, add bell pepper, broccoli florets, snow peas, and julienned carrot. Stir-fry for 4-5 minutes until vegetables are tender-crisp.
- Return cooked turkey to the skillet. Pour in low-sodium chicken or vegetable broth and stir to combine.

- Cook for an additional 2-3 minutes until the broth reduces slightly and coats the turkey and vegetables.
- Sprinkle sliced green onions and sesame seeds over the stir-fry for garnish, if desired.
- Serve the turkey and vegetable stir-fry hot over cooked quinoa or brown rice.

Nutrition Facts (per serving):

- Calories: 320
- Fat: 10g
- Saturated fat: 2g
- Cholesterol: 65mg
- Sodium: 700mg
- Carbohydrate: 22g
- Fiber: 6g
- Sugars: 7g
- Protein: 35g
- Vitamin A: 140%
- Vitamin C: 150%
- Calcium: 10%
- Iron: 15%

Other Ways to Enjoy:

Turkey and Vegetable Lettuce Wraps: Serve the turkey and vegetable stir-fry in large lettuce leaves (such as butter lettuce or romaine) for a low-carb and gluten-free lunch option.

Turkey and Vegetable Grain Bowl: Spoon the turkey and vegetable stir-fry over cooked quinoa, brown rice, or cauliflower rice in a bowl. Top with sliced avocado, chopped cilantro, and a squeeze of lime juice for a satisfying and flavorful grain bowl.

5. Turkey and Avocado Wrap

- Prep Time: 10 mins
- Total Time: 10 mins
- Servings: 2

Ingredients:

- 4 large lettuce leaves (such as romaine or butter lettuce)
- 6 ounces cooked turkey breast, sliced
- 1 avocado, sliced
- 1/2 cup shredded carrots
- 1/2 cup sliced cucumber
- 1/4 cup hummus
- 2 tablespoons sunflower seeds
- Salt and pepper to taste

Directions:

- Lay out the lettuce leaves on a clean work surface.
- Divide the cooked turkey breast evenly among the lettuce leaves.
- Top each lettuce leaf with sliced avocado, shredded carrots, and sliced cucumber.
- Spread hummus evenly over each lettuce leaf.
- Sprinkle sunflower seeds over the fillings.
- Season with salt and pepper to taste.
- Roll up the lettuce leaves tightly to form wraps.
- Slice each wrap in half diagonally.
- Serve immediately and enjoy!

Nutrition Facts (per serving):

- Calories: 320
- Fat: 18g
- Saturated fat: 3g
- Cholesterol: 45mg
- Sodium: 450mg
- Carbohydrate: 18g
- Fiber: 9g
- Sugars: 4g
- Protein: 24g
- Vitamin A: 250%

- Vitamin C: 20%
- Calcium: 8%
- Iron: 15%

Other Ways to Enjoy:

Turkey and Avocado Salad: Chop the lettuce leaves and place them in a large salad bowl. Add sliced turkey breast, avocado, shredded carrots, cucumber, and sunflower seeds. Toss with your favorite vinaigrette dressing for a nutritious salad option.

Turkey and Avocado Lettuce Cups: Use large lettuce leaves as cups and fill them with sliced turkey breast, avocado, shredded carrots, cucumber, and sunflower seeds. Drizzle with a little balsamic glaze or tahini sauce for extra flavor.

Dinner

1. Grilled Lemon Herb Chicken with Roasted Vegetables

- Prep Time: 15 mins
- Total Time: 35 mins
- Servings: 2

Ingredients:

- 2 boneless, skinless chicken breasts

- 2 tablespoons olive oil
- 2 tablespoons lemon juice
- 2 cloves garlic, minced
- 1 teaspoon dried thyme
- 1 teaspoon dried rosemary
- Salt and pepper to taste
- 1 medium zucchini, sliced
- 1 medium yellow squash, sliced
- 1 red bell pepper, sliced
- 1 yellow bell pepper, sliced
- 1 red onion, sliced
- 1 tablespoon balsamic vinegar
- Fresh parsley for garnish (optional)

Directions:

- In a small bowl, whisk together olive oil, lemon juice, minced garlic, dried thyme, dried rosemary, salt, and pepper to create a marinade.
- Place chicken breasts in a shallow dish and pour marinade over them, turning to coat evenly. Allow chicken to marinate in the refrigerator for at least 15 minutes.
- Preheat grill to medium-high heat. Remove chicken from marinade and discard excess marinade. Grill

chicken for 6-7 minutes per side, or until fully cooked and no longer pink in the center.

- While chicken is grilling, preheat oven to 400°F (200°C). In a large bowl, toss sliced zucchini, yellow squash, bell peppers, and red onion with balsamic vinegar, salt, and pepper.
- Spread vegetables evenly on a baking sheet lined with parchment paper. Roast in the preheated oven for 20-25 minutes, or until vegetables are tender and slightly caramelized.
- Once chicken is cooked through and vegetables are roasted, remove from heat.
- Serve grilled lemon herb chicken with roasted vegetables, garnished with fresh parsley if desired.
- Enjoy your nutritious and delicious dinner!

Nutrition Facts (per serving):

- Calories: 380
- Fat: 18g
- Saturated fat: 3g
- Cholesterol: 90mg
- Sodium: 220mg
- Carbohydrate: 15g
- Fiber: 5g
- Sugars: 7g

- Protein: 40g
- Vitamin A: 80%
- Vitamin C: 220%
- Calcium: 10%
- Iron: 15%

Other Ways to Enjoy:

Lemon Herb Chicken Salad: Slice grilled chicken and serve over a bed of mixed greens with roasted vegetables. Drizzle with a lemon vinaigrette dressing for a refreshing salad option.

Lemon Herb Chicken Grain Bowl: Serve sliced grilled chicken with roasted vegetables over cooked quinoa or brown rice. Top with a dollop of Greek yogurt and a sprinkle of chopped fresh herbs for a hearty grain bowl.

2. Baked Salmon with Asparagus and Quinoa

- Prep Time: 10 mins
- Total Time: 30 mins
- Servings: 2

Ingredients:

- 2 salmon fillets (about 6 ounces each)
- 1 tablespoon olive oil
- 1 tablespoon lemon juice

- 2 cloves garlic, minced
- 1 teaspoon dried dill
- Salt and pepper to taste
- 1 bunch asparagus, trimmed
- 1 cup cooked quinoa
- Lemon wedges for serving

Directions:

- Preheat the oven to 400°F (200°C). Line a baking sheet with parchment paper.
- Place the salmon fillets on the prepared baking sheet. Drizzle with olive oil and lemon juice. Sprinkle minced garlic, dried dill, salt, and pepper evenly over the salmon.
- Arrange the trimmed asparagus around the salmon fillets on the baking sheet. Drizzle with a little olive oil and season with salt and pepper.
- Bake in the preheated oven for 15-20 minutes, or until the salmon is cooked through and flakes easily with a fork, and the asparagus is tender.
- While the salmon and asparagus are baking, reheat the cooked quinoa if necessary.
- Divide the cooked quinoa between two plates and top with baked salmon fillets and roasted asparagus.

- Serve with lemon wedges on the side for squeezing over the salmon, if desired.
- Enjoy your nutritious and flavorful dinner!

Nutrition Facts (per serving):

- Calories: 380
- Fat: 18g
- Saturated fat: 3g
- Cholesterol: 90mg
- Sodium: 200mg
- Carbohydrate: 20g
- Fiber: 5g
- Sugars: 3g
- Protein: 36g
- Vitamin A: 20%
- Vitamin C: 25%
- Calcium: 6%
- Iron: 20%

Other Ways to Enjoy:

Salmon and Asparagus Salad: Flake baked salmon and serve over a bed of mixed greens with roasted asparagus. Drizzle with a balsamic vinaigrette dressing for a light and refreshing salad option.

Salmon and Asparagus Stir-Fry: Cut baked salmon into bite-sized pieces and stir-fry with cooked quinoa, roasted asparagus, and your favorite stir-fry sauce for a quick and easy dinner stir-fry. Serve over brown rice or cauliflower rice for a low-carb option.

3. Vegetable Stir-Fry with Tofu

- Prep Time: 15 mins
- Total Time: 25 mins
- Servings: 2

Ingredients:

- 8 ounces extra-firm tofu, drained and cubed
- 2 tablespoons soy sauce (or tamari for gluten-free)
- 1 tablespoon sesame oil
- 1 tablespoon cornstarch
- 1 tablespoon olive oil
- 2 cloves garlic, minced
- 1 teaspoon grated fresh ginger
- 1 bell pepper, sliced
- 1 cup broccoli florets
- 1 carrot, julienned
- 1/2 cup sliced mushrooms
- 1/4 cup sliced green onions
- Cooked brown rice or quinoa for serving

Sauce:

- 2 tablespoons soy sauce
- 1 tablespoon rice vinegar
- 1 tablespoon honey or maple syrup
- 1 teaspoon sesame oil
- 1 teaspoon cornstarch
- 2 tablespoons water

Directions:

- In a bowl, toss cubed tofu with soy sauce, sesame oil, and cornstarch until evenly coated. Set aside to marinate for 10 minutes.
- In a small bowl, whisk together all the sauce ingredients until well combined. Set aside.
- Heat olive oil in a large skillet or wok over medium-high heat. Add minced garlic and grated ginger, and sauté for about 1 minute until fragrant.
- Add marinated tofu to the skillet and cook for 5-7 minutes, stirring occasionally, until tofu is golden and slightly crispy on the edges. Remove tofu from the skillet and set aside.
- In the same skillet, add sliced bell pepper, broccoli florets, julienned carrot, and sliced mushrooms. Stir-fry for 5-7 minutes until vegetables are tender-crisp.

- Return cooked tofu to the skillet, along with sliced green onions. Pour the sauce over the tofu and vegetables, stirring well to coat everything evenly.
- Cook for an additional 1-2 minutes, until the sauce has thickened slightly.
- Serve vegetable stir-fry with tofu over cooked brown rice or quinoa.
- Enjoy your flavorful and satisfying dinner!

Nutrition Facts (per serving, without rice/quinoa):

- Calories: 280
- Fat: 16g
- Saturated fat: 2g
- Cholesterol: 0mg
- Sodium: 1020mg
- Carbohydrate: 22g
- Fiber: 5g
- Sugars: 9g
- Protein: 16g
- Vitamin A: 120%
- Vitamin C: 100%
- Calcium: 15%
- Iron: 20%

Other Ways to Enjoy:

Tofu and Vegetable Lettuce Wraps: Serve the tofu and vegetable stir-fry wrapped in large lettuce leaves for a light and refreshing dinner option.

Tofu and Vegetable Noodle Bowl: Toss the tofu and vegetable stir-fry with cooked soba noodles or rice noodles for a delicious and satisfying noodle bowl. Garnish with chopped peanuts or sesame seeds for added crunch.

4. Mushroom and Spinach Stuffed Bell Peppers

- Prep Time: 15 mins
- Total Time: 45 mins
- Servings: 2

Ingredients:

- 2 large bell peppers, halved and seeds removed
- 1 tablespoon olive oil
- 8 ounces mushrooms, chopped
- 2 cloves garlic, minced
- 2 cups fresh spinach leaves, chopped
- 1/2 cup cooked quinoa
- 1/4 cup grated Parmesan cheese
- Salt and pepper to taste
- Fresh parsley for garnish (optional)

Directions:

- Preheat the oven to 375°F (190°C). Place the halved bell peppers cut side up in a baking dish.
- In a large skillet, heat olive oil over medium heat. Add chopped mushrooms and minced garlic, and sauté for 5-7 minutes until mushrooms are tender and golden brown.
- Add chopped spinach to the skillet and cook for an additional 2-3 minutes until spinach is wilted.
- Remove skillet from heat and stir in cooked quinoa and grated Parmesan cheese. Season with salt and pepper to taste.
- Spoon the mushroom and spinach mixture evenly into each bell pepper half, pressing down gently to pack the filling.
- Cover the baking dish with aluminum foil and bake in the preheated oven for 25-30 minutes, or until the bell peppers are tender.
- Remove foil and bake for an additional 5 minutes to lightly brown the tops of the stuffed peppers.
- Garnish with fresh parsley, if desired, before serving.
- Enjoy your nutritious and flavorful dinner!

Nutrition Facts (per serving):

- Calories: 230
- Fat: 10g

- Saturated fat: 2g
- Cholesterol: 5mg
- Sodium: 280mg
- Carbohydrate: 25g
- Fiber: 6g
- Sugars: 6g
- Protein: 12g
- Vitamin A: 160%
- Vitamin C: 320%
- Calcium: 20%
- Iron: 15%

Other Ways to Enjoy:

Mushroom and Spinach Stuffed Portobello Mushrooms: Instead of bell peppers, use large portobello mushroom caps as the base for stuffing. Bake until mushrooms are tender and filling is heated through.

Mushroom and Spinach Stuffed Zucchini Boats: Cut zucchinis in half lengthwise and scoop out the flesh to create "boats." Fill with the mushroom and spinach mixture, sprinkle with breadcrumbs or additional cheese, and bake until zucchini is tender.

5. Lemon Garlic Shrimp with Zucchini Noodles

- Prep Time: 15 mins

- Total Time: 25 mins
- Servings: 2

Ingredients:

- 8 ounces shrimp, peeled and deveined
- 2 medium zucchinis
- 2 tablespoons olive oil
- 3 cloves garlic, minced
- Zest and juice of 1 lemon
- 1/4 teaspoon red pepper flakes (optional)
- Salt and pepper to taste
- Fresh parsley for garnish (optional)

Directions:

- Use a spiralizer to spiralize the zucchinis into noodles. Set aside.
- Heat 1 tablespoon of olive oil in a large skillet over medium heat. Add minced garlic and cook for 1-2 minutes until fragrant.
- Add shrimp to the skillet and cook for 2-3 minutes per side until pink and cooked through. Remove shrimp from the skillet and set aside.
- In the same skillet, add the remaining olive oil and zucchini noodles. Cook for 2-3 minutes, tossing

occasionally, until zucchini noodles are tender but still slightly crisp.

- Return cooked shrimp to the skillet. Add lemon zest, lemon juice, and red pepper flakes (if using). Toss everything together until evenly combined.
- Season with salt and pepper to taste.
- Garnish with fresh parsley, if desired, before serving.
- Enjoy your light and flavorful dinner!

Nutrition Facts (per serving):

- Calories: 250
- Fat: 14g
- Saturated fat: 2g
- Cholesterol: 150mg
- Sodium: 250mg
- Carbohydrate: 10g
- Fiber: 3g
- Sugars: 5g
- Protein: 20g
- Vitamin A: 15%
- Vitamin C: 45%
- Calcium: 8%
- Iron: 15%

Other Ways to Enjoy:

Lemon Garlic Shrimp Lettuce Wraps: Serve the lemon garlic shrimp and zucchini noodles wrapped in large lettuce leaves for a light and refreshing meal.

Lemon Garlic Shrimp Stir-Fry: Add additional vegetables such as bell peppers, snap peas, and mushrooms to the skillet along with the zucchini noodles for a colorful and nutritious shrimp stir-fry. Serve over cooked brown rice or quinoa for a complete meal.

CHAPTER 5

MEAL PLANNING

21 days meal plan

Day 1:

- Breakfast: Easy Fried Rice
- Lunch: Quinoa Salad with Grilled Chicken
- Dinner: Grilled Lemon Herb Chicken with Roasted Vegetables

Day 2:

- Breakfast: Baked Salmon with Asparagus and Quinoa
- Lunch: Mushroom and Spinach Stuffed Bell Peppers
- Dinner: Lemon Garlic Shrimp with Zucchini Noodles

Day 3:

- Breakfast: Turkey and Avocado Wrap
- Lunch: Vegetable Stir-Fry with Tofu
- Dinner: Mushroom and Spinach Stuffed Bell Peppers

Day 4:

- Breakfast: Grilled Lemon Herb Chicken with Roasted Vegetables

- Lunch: Lemon Garlic Shrimp with Zucchini Noodles
- Dinner: Quinoa Salad with Grilled Chicken

Day 5:

- Breakfast: Baked Salmon with Asparagus and Quinoa
- Lunch: Turkey and Avocado Wrap
- Dinner: Vegetable Stir-Fry with Tofu

Day 6:

- Breakfast: Easy Fried Rice
- Lunch: Mushroom and Spinach Stuffed Bell Peppers
- Dinner: Lemon Garlic Shrimp with Zucchini Noodles

Day 7:

- Breakfast: Quinoa Salad with Grilled Chicken
- Lunch: Vegetable Stir-Fry with Tofu
- Dinner: Grilled Lemon Herb Chicken with Roasted Vegetables

Day 8:

- Breakfast: Baked Salmon with Asparagus and Quinoa
- Lunch: Turkey and Avocado Wrap

- Dinner: Mushroom and Spinach Stuffed Bell Peppers

Day 9:

- Breakfast: Lemon Garlic Shrimp with Zucchini Noodles
- Lunch: Grilled Lemon Herb Chicken with Roasted Vegetables
- Dinner: Quinoa Salad with Grilled Chicken

Day 10:

- Breakfast: Vegetable Stir-Fry with Tofu
- Lunch: Mushroom and Spinach Stuffed Bell Peppers
- Dinner: Lemon Garlic Shrimp with Zucchini Noodles

Day 11:

- Breakfast: Easy Fried Rice
- Lunch: Baked Salmon with Asparagus and Quinoa
- Dinner: Turkey and Avocado Wrap

Day 12:

- Breakfast: Quinoa Salad with Grilled Chicken
- Lunch: Lemon Garlic Shrimp with Zucchini Noodles
- Dinner: Vegetable Stir-Fry with Tofu

Day 13:

- Breakfast: Mushroom and Spinach Stuffed Bell Peppers
- Lunch: Grilled Lemon Herb Chicken with Roasted Vegetables
- Dinner: Baked Salmon with Asparagus and Quinoa

Day 14:

- Breakfast: Turkey and Avocado Wrap
- Lunch: Easy Fried Rice
- Dinner: Lemon Garlic Shrimp with Zucchini Noodles

Day 15:

- Breakfast: Vegetable Stir-Fry with Tofu
- Lunch: Quinoa Salad with Grilled Chicken
- Dinner: Mushroom and Spinach Stuffed Bell Peppers

Day 16:

- Breakfast: Baked Salmon with Asparagus and Quinoa
- Lunch: Turkey and Avocado Wrap
- Dinner: Grilled Lemon Herb Chicken with Roasted Vegetables

Day 17:

- Breakfast: Lemon Garlic Shrimp with Zucchini Noodles
- Lunch: Mushroom and Spinach Stuffed Bell Peppers
- Dinner: Quinoa Salad with Grilled Chicken

Day 18:

- Breakfast: Easy Fried Rice
- Lunch: Vegetable Stir-Fry with Tofu
- Dinner: Baked Salmon with Asparagus and Quinoa

Day 19:

- Breakfast: Turkey and Avocado Wrap
- Lunch: Lemon Garlic Shrimp with Zucchini Noodles
- Dinner: Grilled Lemon Herb Chicken with Roasted Vegetables

Day 20:

- Breakfast: Mushroom and Spinach Stuffed Bell Peppers
- Lunch: Quinoa Salad with Grilled Chicken
- Dinner: Vegetable Stir-Fry with Tofu

Day 21:

- Breakfast: Baked Salmon with Asparagus and Quinoa

- Lunch: Easy Fried Rice
- Dinner: Lemon Garlic Shrimp with Zucchini Noodles

CHAPTER 6

SHOPPING GUIDE

How to Shop for Epi Diet Foods

Plan Your Meals:

- Before heading to the grocery store, plan your meals for the week. Consider incorporating a variety of fruits, vegetables, lean proteins, whole grains, and healthy fats into your meal plan.

- Create a shopping list based on your meal plan to ensure you have all the ingredients you need.

Read Labels:

- When shopping for packaged foods, carefully read the ingredient lists and nutrition labels.

- Look for products that contain whole, unprocessed ingredients and avoid those with added sugars, artificial additives, and preservatives.

- Check for hidden sugars, unhealthy fats, and excessive sodium content in products.

Choose Whole Foods:

- Prioritize whole foods such as fresh fruits and vegetables, lean proteins (e.g., poultry, fish, tofu), whole grains (e.g., quinoa, brown rice, oats), and healthy fats (e.g., olive oil, avocado, nuts).

- Opt for organic produce and locally sourced foods whenever possible to minimize exposure to pesticides and support sustainable farming practices.

Select Lean Proteins:

- Choose lean sources of protein, such as skinless poultry, fish, tofu, beans, and legumes.
- Avoid processed meats and high-fat cuts of meat, which may contain unhealthy additives and excessive saturated fats.

Prioritize Healthy Fats:

- Select sources of healthy fats, such as olive oil, avocado, nuts, and seeds.
- Avoid products containing hydrogenated oils and trans fats, which can negatively impact heart health.

Shop for Whole Grains:

- Choose whole grain products, including whole wheat bread, brown rice, quinoa, oats, and whole grain pasta, over refined grains.

- Look for products labeled "100% whole grain" or "whole wheat" to ensure they contain the entire grain kernel.

Minimize Processed Foods:

- Minimize your intake of processed foods, including packaged snacks, sugary beverages, and convenience meals.
- Focus on cooking meals from scratch using whole, nutrient-dense ingredients.

Budget-Friendly Tips:

- Plan your grocery trips to avoid impulse purchases and minimize food waste.
- Compare prices of similar products and look for sales, discounts, and coupons to save money.
- Consider buying staple items such as grains, beans, and nuts in bulk to reduce costs over time.

Reading Labels and Identifying Epi Diet-Friendly Products

Scan the Ingredient List:

- Look for whole, unprocessed foods listed as primary ingredients. These include fruits, vegetables, whole grains, lean proteins, and healthy fats.

- Avoid products with added sugars, artificial additives, preservatives, and highly processed ingredients.
- Be cautious of hidden sources of sugar, such as high fructose corn syrup, dextrose, and maltose.
- Check for unhealthy fats like trans fats and hydrogenated oils, and opt for products with healthy fats such as olive oil, avocado oil, and nuts.

Check the Nutrition Facts:

- Pay attention to serving sizes and the number of servings per container to accurately assess nutritional content.
- Monitor calories, fat, sodium, carbohydrates, fiber, and protein per serving. Aim for balanced meals with moderate amounts of each nutrient.
- Choose products with lower sodium content and opt for reduced-sodium or no-salt-added options.
- Prioritize foods high in fiber to promote satiety and digestive health.

Look for Whole Grains:

- Choose whole grain products such as brown rice, quinoa, oats, whole wheat bread, and whole grain pasta.

- Avoid refined grains and products made with white flour or enriched flour.

Select Lean Proteins:

- Opt for lean sources of protein such as skinless poultry, fish, tofu, tempeh, legumes, and lentils.
- Avoid processed meats like sausages, bacon, and deli meats, which often contain added sodium and unhealthy fats.

Choose Healthy Fats:

- Look for sources of healthy fats such as olive oil, avocado, nuts, seeds, and fatty fish like salmon and mackerel.
- Avoid products containing trans fats and limit saturated fats.

Consider Organic and Locally Sourced Options:

- Whenever possible, choose organic produce and locally sourced foods to minimize exposure to pesticides and support sustainable farming practices.

CHAPTER 7

CONCLUSION

In conclusion, adopting the Epi Diet involves making mindful choices about the foods we consume, prioritizing whole, nutrient-dense ingredients while avoiding processed and unhealthy options. By understanding the principles of the Epi Diet and learning how to shop for Epi Diet-friendly foods, individuals can embark on a journey towards better health and well-being.

Reading labels and identifying Epi Diet-friendly products is essential when grocery shopping. This involves scanning ingredient lists for whole, unprocessed foods, checking nutrition facts for balanced macronutrient profiles, and selecting products high in fiber and low in added sugars and unhealthy fats. Choosing whole grains, lean proteins, and healthy fats, while minimizing processed foods and sodium intake, can help individuals adhere to the Epi Diet guidelines.

Furthermore, budget-friendly tips such as meal planning, buying in-season produce, purchasing staple items in bulk, and utilizing coupons and discounts can help individuals shop for Epi Diet foods without breaking the bank. Prioritizing organic and locally sourced options whenever possible supports not only personal health but also environmental sustainability.

In essence, by adopting the strategies discussed for shopping for Epi Diet foods and incorporating them into everyday life, individuals can make informed decisions that promote optimal health, vitality, and longevity. The journey towards better nutrition and well-being starts with the choices we make at the grocery store and extends to every meal we enjoy.

Made in the USA
Las Vegas, NV
28 September 2024

95922361R00059